Last Resort Sugar Detox Guide
by Michael Collins

TABLE OF CONTENTS

INTRODUCTION

MY STORY, OR "WHO THE HECK IS THIS GUY?"

THE LIES THAT SUGAR ADDICTS TELL THEMSELVES

THE LONG-TERM RISKS OF SUGAR ADDICTION

EASY DOES IT

Sugar Addicts Are Extremely Hard on Themselves

Why Beating Yourself Up Doesn't Work

Contrary Action: Being Easy on Yourself

Being Easy on Yourself is Not a Free Pass to Not Do the Work

BINGE EATING AND SUGAR ADDICTION

Checklist for Binge Eating Disorder

AWARENESS, ACCEPTANCE, ACTION

Acceptance Always Precedes Change

Always Check with Your Doctor First

YOUR GAME PLAN FOR A "QUICK WIN"

Preparing yourself.

Take as long as you need.

How long you detox is up to you.

Preparing your family.

This detox is for YOU.

Preparing your workplace.

Drawing Your Line in The Sand -

Choosing Your Day and Preparing Your Environment.

"Feel the guilt and DO IT Anyway."

ADDICTION AND CRAVING AND WILLPOWER, OH MY!

Addiction: No One Wants To Admit To This Ugly Word

The Power of Sugar and Flour

Cravings

Volume as a Trigger

THE MYTH OF WILLPOWER

Dependency Can't Be Controlled By Willpower Alone
Abstinence

WHAT TO EXPECT

The Benefits of Sugar and Flour Abstinence are Vast

Cravings will Subside with Abstinence

A Bonus Side Note and a Vision of the Future about the Growling Stomach

WITHDRAWALS

What to Expect with Withdrawals

How To Cope With Withdrawals

Day-by-day Outline of Walking Through and Managing Withdrawal

FOOD PLAN FOR RECOVERY

Benefits of Following the Food Plan

NSFW: No Sugar, Flour & Wheat

JOURNALING: A TOOL FOR SUCCESS

The Importance of Rigorous Honesty

BODY IMAGE

Acceptance at All Weights

SELF-CARE AND EXERCISE: WORKING OUT AND WORKING WITHIN

Examples of Self-Care

EXERCISE: IT'S NOT WHAT YOU THINK

How Exercise Helps in Recovering From Sugar Addiction

How to Create a Realistic Exercise Plan

MEDITATION

Benefits of Meditation

How To Meditate

YOU CAN'T DO THIS ALONE: OUR SUPPORT GROUP

Successful People Never Do It Alone

A Word On 12-Step Programs

CONCLUSION

INTRODUCTION

Welcome to The Last Resort Sugar Detox from the Original SugarAddiction.com

Congratulations! You've just taken the first step in the process of helping yourself out of the sugar prison you have been trapped in for years or even decades. It takes a lot of courage to look this, or any, habit or dependency in the face and make a commitment to change.

We hope that within this book you will find understanding, compassion, guidance, and, most of all, hope.

Please take comfort in the fact that you are not alone.

We take our stewardship of SugarAddiction.com very seriously and strive to offer everyone who visits our website the very best information, community, and support to assist people in the process of gaining control over sugar and your life.

As the science around sugar and how it affects the body increases, almost daily, we know that this topic will be of great interest to folks worldwide for many years to come.

Having been there ourselves, we know exactly how you feel. We are not a boot camp. We are not a diet. We are not a fad. We are here to bring you cutting-edge information and support for a confusing topic that is causing immense pain to some - worldwide.

You've already taken the first step by seeking out help. This book is intended to walk you through the process of change and recovery. We want you to live a happy and fulfilled life, free from the physical and emotional chains of eating too much sugar, and we can help you achieve this goal.

Step two, if you haven't already done so, is to join the private Sugar Detox Daily Support Group on Facebook.

Just request entrance and our administrators will approve you if you've purchased or downloaded this book.

My Story, or "Who the Heck is this Guy?"

It all started with caffeine…

I remember working in restaurants and bars to pay my way through college, and as the bartender, all the employees had to come through me to get their drinks.

The drinks were free - so a strange dynamic developed as folks could drink unlimited amounts and cost was not a factor.

I started to notice a strange observational phenomena: it didn't matter if it was the 16 year old busboy or the 60 year old cook—the folks that drank the most caffeine developed dark circles under their eyes, and it was relative as to amount. The people with the largest habits had the darkest circles under their eyes.

That awareness began a lifetime of personal exploration into the substances we put into our bodies.

It also led to my personal recovery from alcohol and drug addiction (another book—currently in the works), flour and sugar dependency, and even a few more.

Early in my recovery from drugs and alcohol I started to notice that caffeine and sugar were present at a lot of the support groups. Every meeting and every event was a sugar and caffeine smorgasbord.

Then I noticed that all the new folks started to pack on what is commonly called in college "the freshman 15" - myself included.

Addiction professionals will tell you about "substituting one drug for another," and it seemed very obvious to me that everyone was substituting sugar and caffeine for their drugs of choice. The obvious also happened, the freshman 15 got much larger for many, many folks.

When I would talk about flour, sugar and caffeine, people took to calling me the "weird addiction" specialist. They weren't really interested in my thoughts and theories as long as I was staying clean and sober from what they considered "harder drugs" and alcohol.

As my recovery advanced, I eventually quit caffeine, and then sugar and then flour much in the way I describe here in the book. The only difference was, even though I was surrounded by addiction-savvy people, my journey was pretty much alone.

The one thing, along with years of research and trial and error, that cemented my beliefs in this subject was the pregnancy of my wife and the birth of my children—identical twin boys. By some miracle my wife bought into my beliefs and vowed with me not to eat flour or sugar or ingest caffeine during the pregnancy.

Just as a point of interest, for the moms or moms to be, she delivered just shy of 14 pounds of baby(s), 6.9 ounces each, and she gained a grand total of 20 pounds during the pregnancy.

We then raised the boys without sugar, flour or caffeine for the first six years of their lives. After that, about once a month, we would allow them to eat it at other children's birthdays but never at home. Yes, it was crazy hard convincing and educating family members, school officials, and babysitters, but I believe with all my heart that it created much healthier children.

A quick story about withdrawals from sugar and the reactions it has in the body involving the kids.

My mother once told me I was a "perfect angel" as a kid. My response, like everyone who would hear that - gosh thanks mom! But she didn't stop there. She continued to tell me a story about falling asleep.

Apparently almost every time I would fall asleep my hair would get soaked with sweat and I would form this perfect little halo in my pillow! She thought nothing of it, she just thought it was cute.

So remembering that story I always watched for the little halo on my kids. It never came. Until that one day, I remember it like it was yesterday. We were at a roller skating rink for yet another child's birthday party. The cake and ice cream came out. Both my boys, at the same time craned their necks toward us as if to say "can we please? Can we please?"

We just gave in. Six years of a battle with friends, parents, school administrators and our own families just seemed like too much (we regained our resolve the next day).

I know you can guess what I'm going to say next though.

-- So that evening I went into the boy's room and guess what I see for the first time? You guessed it - two perfect little halos and soaking wet hair. My boys were in sugar detox! (More on this in the withdrawals section)

I consider myself a smart enough guy folks, but my boys are rocket scientist smart. One of them got a perfect score on his original SATs and his brother missed just one question. My scores and those of their mom, were much closer to average. I believe that their brains just developed better because they were free of sugar and the science is just now bearing that out.

On the other end of the spectrum, my parents are both in the early stages of Alzheimer's, which now starting to be called "Type 3 Diabetes." I can't necessarily prove to you that sugar caused this, but my dear mother has been a sugar junkie her entire life and my father joined her after he slowed down his drinking. There are studies now that have speculated on this.

I believe that one day, in the advancement of human history, 200 years from now we'll look back and say things like "Did you know they used to give sugar to children?" Much like we say now "Did you know they used to put cocaine in Coca Cola?"

For most of human history people have come together as a community or tribe to pass on information and provide support in order to tackle things that we "know" but can't seem to "do" without help.

This book and SugarAddiction.com serve to continue that tradition. I hope you'll join us so that we can help each other to change your life and the lives of the millions of people affected by this terrible dependency.

If you still have any doubt, after going online and researching a little about sugar, researching books, finding this one and ordering it - that you may have an issue with sugar - feel free to take our very short, yet very effective, free sugar quiz right here...

THE LIES THAT SUGAR ADDICTS TELL THEMSELVES

Like anyone suffering from a bad habit, dependency or addiction over which they seem to have little or no control, people with even a mild sugar dependency have a constant script that runs through their head on a loop that criticizes, scolds, and humiliates them.

That inner voice causes them to eat sugar compulsively just to shut it up, but that moment of relief is fleeting—and the pleasure in eating usually has more to do with quieting the internal monologue than the sugar itself. Most, if not all, of what this inner critic is telling you is a big pack of lies.

Sugar increases the production of dopamine, which stimulates the reward system of pleasure. This stimulation is often short-lived and leaves us wanting more.

Here are the most common lies that sugar addicts tell themselves:

- Eating sugar will make me feel better.
- This is the last time.
- Since I can hide it from other people, it's not really a big deal.
- As long as I only binge eat on the weekends, it's not out of control.
- I just did XYZ—I deserve to celebrate!
- I'll start that diet/exercise program tomorrow.
- I'll exercise for two hours to compensate for the box of donuts I just ate.
- I am only loveable at a certain weight/nobody loves me/I'm completely unlovable.
- If I can't have a perfect relationship with food then it's not worth even trying.
- Since I don't eat SUGAR all the time, IT isn't really that bad.
- I just need to have stronger willpower.
- Something is very wrong with me.
- I'm a failure.
- I have a successful career, so this means that I don't have a real problem.

Find out if you are a sugar addict. Take the quiz here!

THE LONG-TERM RISKS OF SUGAR ADDICTION

Many people over-satiate themselves now and again—we all know that uncomfortable feeling of eating too much—but regularly doing this long-term puts you at risk for health problems. According to Nancy Appleton, the grand dame of sugar educators, these are some of the physical consequences of over consuming sugar (her list is actually over 140):

- high blood pressure
- high cholesterol
- heart disease
- type 2 diabetes
- gallbladder disease
- sleep apnea or insomnia
- edema
- kidney disease

- degenerative arthritis
- infertility
- some types of cancer
- irritable bowel syndrome (IBS)
- fibromyalgia

The good news is that the sooner you get help, the better your chances of recovery.

EASY DOES IT

As you read this book, I want you to be kind to yourself. We find that sugar addicts are remarkably hard on themselves. Really hard. In fact, downright mean.

One thing we have found, time and time again, is that "beating yourself up" (yes, a medical term) is of absolutely no help.

Look at it this way: if beating yourself up worked, you'd be A-OK right now.

The thing to keep in mind is that you didn't get here in one day and you won't walk out of here tomorrow. But if you make a personal commitment to caring for yourself first and foremost, then you stand a much better chance of recovering than if you constantly berate yourself.

Beating yourself up stops today.

[Listen here to the affirmations now to stop beating yourself up!](#)

Sugar Addicts Are Extremely Hard on Themselves

People who qualify as a sugar addict or as a binge eater tend to be unusually hard on themselves. This is not only very destructive, **but may in fact have been a catalyst for this symptomatic behavior in the first place**. Self-care is just as important as discipline—maybe even more so—because you won't overcome any disorder if you can't care for and about yourself in every way.

Later in this book we will be instructing you to do small, kind things for yourself. At first they will seem ridiculous (you might even feel like that *Saturday Night Live* character Stuart Smalley!).

But here's the key: do them anyway. Self-care is the core, the very foundation, of helping yourself walk through and out of this hell and it cannot be underestimated. Just as your destructive behavior developed over time, you'll need to be patient with yourself as you practice being kind to yourself.

What follows is a comprehensive plan to change your behavior around sugar and food.

This plan may sound daunting or frightening, but countless others have faced the same challenge and been victorious.

You can do it, too! You'll have to do the work, and it won't always be easy, but it *is* possible and it is imperative for your health—physically and emotionally.

You've already cleared the first hurdle by reading this book so far, so give yourself a pat on the back for that. As far as we're concerned, you are already beginning to triumph over sugar.

If you'd like a deeper look into what to expect on this journey check out a clip from our video course, which is a compliment to this book, entitled "What to Expect." It's FREE to check out right here.

Why Beating Yourself Up Doesn't Work

"God, you're so stupid!"

"What a big, fat loser you are."

"You never do anything right."

"Do you know how grotesque you look right now?"

"No wonder no one loves you."

Do these phrases sound terrible to you? Of course they do! Yet we say them to ourselves all the time. If our friends treated us the way we treat ourselves, chances are we would walk away from them.

So the next time you berate yourself, listen to the words your inner critic is saying and then imagine saying the exact same thing to your best friend. Isn't that a heartbreaking image? In many cases, it would even be considered verbal abuse.

So why are we so willing to treat ourselves this way?

Believe it or not, this inner critic is just doing what it believes is necessary to protect us and ensure that we are safe. It comes down to basic survival skills in the face of danger—or in many cases, perceived danger. The biological "fight or flight" response that we feel when threatened (whether the threat is real or imaginary) is designed to ignore the pain, danger or risk of death and do what is necessary to motivate us into surviving at any costs.

Just as beating someone else up, physically or emotionally, never works, beating ourselves up is also futile. Let me repeat this very important concept: *if beating yourself up actually worked, you'd have stopped using sugar years ago.*

Beating yourself up never works.

Contrary Action: Being Easy on Yourself

So if beating ourselves up isn't the answer, what is? Simple: loving ourselves. Having compassion for ourselves. Understanding that we have simply been doing the best that we could given the circumstances—and by circumstances, we mean not fully comprehending the severity of our disorder and not having a place to seek help.

Contrary action is any action that is, quite simply, different from what you'd normally do. The idea behind this concept is that you have been making decisions from the part of your mind that may be unhealthy or untrained, so if you want to make healthy choices, you can't rely on this part of your mind.

You must allow your mind to make its default choice, and then do the opposite. And yes, it will feel unnatural and uncomfortable and wrong. At first. But eventually, as you get used to this new dynamic, making healthy choices will become second nature to you and feel more comfortable.

The first contrary action we are going to ask you to perform is to be easy on yourself. Cut yourself some slack. Be proud that you have sought help. Take a deep breath.

Being Easy on Yourself is Not a Free Pass to Not Do the Work

Many people cannot fathom being easy on themselves because doing so feels like they're not taking their situation seriously. They're afraid that they or, more importantly, others will assume that they are condoning their sugar addiction.

So let's be clear here. Being easy on yourself isn't a free pass.

It doesn't mean that you don't take this disorder seriously. It doesn't mean that you get to avoid doing the work. It doesn't mean you condone your behavior and invite more of the same into your life.

Being easy on yourself just means that you are human, you deserve to be loved, and you get to practice compassion for this vastly serious disorder from which you are suffering.

If you're a video watcher, instead of a reader, you might have interest in my interview on The Kick Sugar Summit with my co-host and co-founder. It really mirrors this book and complements it in many ways. The interview will give you a great overview of the book and you can always refer back to the book for the nuts and bolts specifics. [Watch it here for free](#)

BINGE EATING AND SUGAR ADDICTION

A related and sometimes co-occurring malady, binge eating, sometimes affects sugar addicts.

Binge Eating is not just overeating, having cravings now and again, indulging in dessert during the holidays or on special occasions, or eating too much when you are hungry.

The typical binge eater is very similar to the alcoholic in that once she's had the first "drink" (cookie, donut, chip, etc.) she spirals out of control and can't stop until the whole thing is gone.

He may sneak into the kitchen in the middle of the night to devour an entire carton of ice cream while standing up in the light of the refrigerator. She is usually plotting out her next rendezvous with her food of choice, including which store or café she will stop at to stock up. She may turn down invites from people, go home early to seek comfort in a bag of cookies, or feel resentful of people who can stop eating after one piece, handful, or bite.

This cycle repeats itself again and again, with vicious bouts of guilt, self-hatred, despair, and hopelessness. The binge eater may or may not promise herself that this time will really be the last time, but because of her powerlessness over this condition, it never is—even as she gains weight, suffers from health problems, or damages relationships.

Binge eating is compulsive and it's emotional. But at its core, it has a very strong relationship to sugar addiction as most people binge on sugary products at least partially. More about binge eating here

Checklist for Binge Eating Disorder

Everyone occasionally overeats—especially during the holidays, when they're under stress, or in social situations. But consuming large quantities of food or being overweight does not necessarily make you a binge eater.

Professionals agree that in order to be diagnosed as a binge eater, a person has to exhibit the symptoms listed below at least once a week for more than three months:

- Overwhelming feelings that you cannot control what you are eating or how much you are eating
- Recurring incidents of eating very large amounts of food in one sitting
- Eating much faster than you normally would (in front of other people)
- Eating to the point where you are uncomfortably full
- Eating an excessive amount of food even though you don't feel hungry physically

- Recurring incidents of eating alone due to embarrassment at the amount of food you are eating
- Overwhelming feelings of shame, guilt, disgust or depression because of what you have just done
- Massive variations in your weight
- Low or no self-esteem
- Noticeable decrease in sexual energy/desire
- The desire to try various diets

If any of these symptoms apply to you, please do not feel bad. Awareness is the first step to finding a solution to any problem in life. The fact that you are reading this book shows that you are a smart individual who cares enough about yourself

to take responsibility for and seek positive change in your life. You are much more than merely a group of symptoms, so go easy on yourself as you continue reading this book. Compassion for yourself is just as important as courage; in fact, they are synonymous.

To better assess if you might be at risk for binge eating, take the free binge eating quiz here.

AWARENESS, ACCEPTANCE, ACTION

Chances are, if you have tried to stop eating sugar and were unsuccessful at it, it's because you attempted to jump straight to the solution. You may have thrown out all the tempting food in your kitchen. You likely went on a diet. You might have even tried socializing only with people for whom food wasn't a problem. You bribed yourself with a reward if you managed to not eat sugar for a week.

But before you even think about the solution, you must be truly and fully aware of the problem.

Otherwise you're just in denial, and being in denial makes you susceptible to being sucked back into the problem again. Being fully aware of the issue means understanding how you came to binge eat or use lots of sugar in the first place, what's going on at a deeper level. (It is not really about sugar)

Only when we've become sincerely aware of our situation can we move on to acceptance. This concept is often a difficult one to embrace because, as we mentioned earlier, most people mistake accepting a situation for condoning it.

Let's clear this up right now. To condone is to approve of something that is considered wrong and allow it to continue. To accept something is simply to agree with reality. All we're asking you to do is to agree with reality, which may sound something like: "I may have a slight sugar dependency" or "I have an unhealthy relationship to sugar."

Once we're aware of our problem and accept that we have this problem, only then can we effectively take the actions necessary to solve the problem.

Acceptance Always Precedes Change

A final word on acceptance. It is a fundamental truth that acceptance always precedes change. Being able to accept yourself, your struggles, your past, your emotions, and your setbacks—not to mention your successes, your future, your self-worth, and your happiness—is the key that unlocks the door to recovery. Stop fighting yourself. Stop fighting reality. Accept and love yourself just the way you are, even when it seems ridiculous, uncomfortable, and counter-intuitive. In fact, *especially* when it seems ridiculous, uncomfortable, and counter-intuitive.

Always Check with Your Doctor First

Before starting any physical change (diet, exercise), always check with your doctor first to ensure that any existing or potential health problems aren't triggered. The Mayo Clinic suggests checking with your doctor if any of the following apply:

- You have heart disease

- You have asthma or lung disease
- You have diabetes or kidney disease
- You have arthritis

It's doubtful that many docs will have too much of an issue with you taking a break from sugar but please ask first.

YOUR GAME PLAN FOR A "QUICK WIN"

There are a few other things you need to do before we get started on the nuts and bolts.

There are different preparations you need to take so as to make your detox as successful as possible.

...And there are different people that need to be prepared. It's not just you!

You need to prepare yourself sure but you also need to prepare your family, your friends and your workmates. This will truly take a village.

Preparing yourself.

The first and most important step in preparing yourself is to determine your WHY!!

Why are you wanting to reduce or eliminate sugar in your life?

This step may take some soul searching but it is absolutely mandatory, at this juncture, that you sit for a minute and ask yourself WHY you want to quit sugar.

Sit with a pen and paper or at a new Word Doc and just list the reasons you want to quit or control sugar. No thought just list for now - do it fast and list as many as you can.

Is it for weight loss?

Is it because of a diabetes diagnosis?

Other health issues?

Once your finished listing all the reasons then form a "WHY" statement just for you. See below for an example.

Once you've determined your why you need to quit - write it down. Put it on a 3x5 card, get it laminated and put it in your wallet. Tape it to your bathroom mirror. Make it your screensaver on your phone, tablet, laptop and desktop!

In short do whatever it takes to see this mantra every day.

So let's say your "why" is the following:

"I need to quit sugar to stem the tide of this yearly weight gain, finally get healthy again and to be able to live see my kids get married and have children"

That's a solid why. It tells you exactly why you need to push through the difficult times.

Once you settle on the reason why it will help if you do this exercise.

Sit quietly and visualize your ideal self without sugar.

- Close your eyes and **see and feel** exactly what your life would be like when you were in complete control of your sugar.
- See your new body at your goal weight.
- See and feel how that feels, how you feel in the world.
- See yourself being able to say a simple and polite no to sugar and mean it this time.

See yourself celebrating one year off sugar and actually look at your NEW self in the mirror.

This little exercise seems silly but it is the basis of almost all personal and self development programs.

Don't worry there is lots of actual nuts and bolts, and honestly a little hard work, to come but for now I just want you to tap into your imagination and see your ideal future.

Take as long as you need.

"Borrow from the beauty of the future to enroll yourself in the activities of today"

Then set a goal.

How long you detox is up to you.

We suggest 30 days but anything more than one day will help. We will describe an entire 30 day detox but everyone is just a little different.
Our facebook group will help you be accountable. Join here!

This a self paced program. We're always here to help but eventually you need to be making your own decisions around sugar.

Preparing your family.

If you live with others they are going to be intimately involved in this journey.

If your kids are young and you have the support of your spouse then this will go much more smoothly.

But regardless of your circumstances this is very possible for anyone, in any situation. Do NOT use your family or living situation as an excuse.

We have success stories from moms of four kids and women who live alone. Only you can determine your destiny.

But…

You need to tell your family what you're up to.

Trying this in a vacuum just won't work. If there is pushback then you just need to learn to deal with it right now. (Don't worry we can help with that, learning to have these conversations with confidence may be one of the most important skills we can teach you)

Tell them you plan on stopping sugar for a set period of time. Tell them they don't have to change anything and MEAN IT.

The first step in all this is to help yourself.

Now if your family finds that this is something you all want to do as a team then more power to you but DO NOT make this a requirement for them or for you!

Put your own oxygen mask on first as they say on the airlines. Once you've mastered the sugar then you can help others.

One of the Catch-22's of this process is that you will need to clean the house out of sugar. Which may or may not be tricky depending on your family's habits. But we'll show you a way to deal with that below.

This detox is for YOU.

We have entire programs devoted to our graduates helping others and we'd love to have you as an instructor. But the first requirement is that they master the sugar for themselves.

You need to be a little selfish for a time. For most of our clients this is actually one of the hardest parts of the entire process. Taking time for themselves. Not buying "treats" for the family. (They get enough outside the home believe me)

But please think of this just the same way the airlines do. You truly can not help anyone until you are first safe on the other side.

Preparing your workplace.

At work you can be a little more stealth and stay hidden under the radar. It really depends on how tight knit your work group is. If it's like family and there are lots of "sugar sharing" events then you'll need to come clean.

The same applies as above with your family.

Do not get into the "recruiting people to join you" business just yet.

Let folks make their own decisions. If they ask you, and only if they ask you, send them a link to this book on Amazon and let the rest go - for now.

Seriously just tell them that this is something you need to do and ask them to please support you.

Hugely Important Note

This "coming out" - this explaining your new behaviors and actions to your family and others is quite possibly the THE most important part of your journey.

Your family, nuclear and extended, workmates and the general public.

You'll need to practice.

As I write this we just got a post on our private forum from a woman who has been off sugar for more than five months. She was having dinner with a friend who had a terrible loss. When the dinner ended and the friend wanted a treat my client just couldn't bear to bring up all "the sugar stuff" by saying "no you go ahead" and instead she joined her.

She caught herself early and didn't go on a binge, so all is well, but early in your sugar detox these conversations are critical!

- I mean critical.
- You have to have them.
- You need to stay strong.
- You need to refer to your why to get through the tougher social interactions.
- It's soooo… important!
- Having a supportive group of friends will help make this easier.

Drawing Your Line in The Sand -

Choosing Your Day and Preparing Your Environment.

Ok, once you have mentally prepared yourself and the others in your life it's time to draw your line in the sand and choose a day to start.

We'll go over the exact sugar withdrawal symptoms later but suffice it to say there will be a few rocky days at first and you need to choose wisely as to WHEN to begin.

We find that people have the most success when they have the least stress and the most time to rest and pamper themselves a little for the first few days.

That's why we suggest a long weekend. Not a holiday where there will be activity and social events but one you create and can just hibernate for three or four days.

Take a personal day on a Friday or a Monday. Do it at a time where you can just have the time for you. Light family or social obligations and nothing stressful. My mom used to call it - "puttering around the house."

You're going to want to rest, read or watch movies, eat well, exercise mildly and generally pamper yourself with massages etc.

This YOUR time. Which, as I mentioned before, will be harder for you to take than the actual stuff you need to do. You'll feel a little guilty at first...

"Feel the guilt and DO IT Anyway."

You must stem this sugar flow into your body.

You must get a handle on this. We have decades of experience with this and it really is worth it!

If you've been able to wrangle a Friday off and are ready then your start date will be Thursday morning.

Your first day is a weird "grace" day, so work that day shouldn't be too hard. You may have a slight headache and be a little irritable and tired by day's end but you'll make it to an early bedtime and have three solid days to add to your first day.

And if possibly you slip it will be small and you still have three solid days to work with before it's back to everyday life.

I suggest cleaning out your entire house of any sugar products on Wednesday night.

And I do mean everything.

Of course all the obvious candy, cookies and ice cream but also all ketchups, mayonnaises, salad dressings and hidden sugar type products as well.

Your mind will delude you during this process into thinking this is an OK thing to have. "Just a little".

But it never works.

This sounds like a lot, and a bit drastic, but take my word if you're serious this step is vitally important.

It provides you a clear line in the sand and a cathartic "ceremony" from which to start.

Plus if you quit it gets expensive to replace all that stuff and we need to put small obstacles in our way. This is a simple and cheap one.

Physical vs Emotional Detox.

Before I walk you through exactly what to expect on days one through thirty I want to stress something. I want split apart the physical detox from the emotional or mental detox.

This concept is key to our long-term success with or clients.

Every other detox out there focuses on the FOOD.

They all have elaborate food plans and recipe books. Their emails are filled with "sugar-free" desserts and such.

While you need to adjust your diet from the one you are currently eating, my guess is you already know that.

You even know what to eat.

Our average client has been in OVER TEN different programs and has read and tried that many diets.

Most are well meaning folks who are correct in what they describe. Low carb, no white stuff etc.

The problem is diets don't work.

We all know this.

And if they work for a short time and folks get with the program of the "correct" food - over 98+ percent of the time they fall back to a place that was worse than they started. The facts and the studies are very clear on this.

Let me be very clear.

Down below you will find EXACTLY what to eat. We definitely don't leave that out.

Some people have never been exposed to the correct food plan and we want you to have that and follow it. But my guess is you're here because you have, like most of our clients, quite literally tried everything!

What isn't so well known, or known at all, is what we call the emotional detox.

Followed by the emotional and mental re-configuring necessary to be successful long term.

You need to literally rewire your brain back to it's

factory settings.

As with most things in life - this is a mental game.

I'm saying you can not "think" your way out of this - you can't.

What I'm asking you to do is suspend judgment for the next one day, one week up to thirty day period and to see if your emotions are one of the keys to unlocking your long-term success.

To pay as much attention to how you FEEL as to what you eat or don't eat or how many sit ups you do…

Once the sugar is removed, if you've ever struggled with this before then SOMETHING is going to happen. Something is going to change, and that something is going to feel like your mind and emotions are going a little haywire…

If you don't track it - if you don't understand it - if you don't deal with it….

You are bound to repeat it.

- You will be emotional.

- You may be inexplicably weepy.

- You'll be angry for no reason.

- Sad for no reason.

- You'll be depressed a little. Not to worry it's not a mental issue it's a physical withdrawal symptom.

- The stress will feel unbearable at times.

- When the only thing you can think of is your go-to sweet. - That should be the biggest clue ever!

If you want check out a quick video on "Sugar Cravings and Your Emotions, Physical detox vs the emotional detox" just look here.

What I'm trying to make clear here is that everything you've been taught about success on sugar detoxes and diets is wrong.

At the very least they have left out the one or two parts that are **the golden keys to the golden lock** - your emotional state and the transition to a new method of coping with everyday stress without sugar.

So how do we change that?

At first, we don't. We manage it. We understand it. Then we change it.

None of this work can begin until you are first clean of sugar.

Now the time DURING the initial detox is super important because the crazy emotional ups and downs if they are not understood and dealt with, can stop our forward progress in its tracks.

We've all experienced it...

We try to quit sugar, or do any diet, for a few days, a week or longer and it's rough during the withdrawals.

But the main stumbling block seems to end up at the cravings.

Those darn cravings.

It's like another person inside us.

We've decided to quit or take a break from the stuff but our mind, even our body "feels" like it "wants" something sweet.

It's hard to even explain to another person but anyone who's had the feeling knows what I'm talking about.

You know, where your mind thinks about it and your mouth can feel the sweetness and the texture hours before you ever ingest the stuff.

I venture to say our entire body can feel, think about and anticipate the little "rush" we get, the little pick me up.

We're a little tired, maybe a little blue or maybe just a little bored. And we know a soda or a candy bar will knock that feeling right out for a few minutes so we can finish our work or just nod out after.

It's insidious I tell you.

So how do we beat the ol' sugar demons?

Well everybody says we detox off the stuff.

That getting the stuff out of our system will lessen or eliminate the cravings.

But what happens when that doesn't work?

When you've quit for weeks or months but you still have cravings that end up derailing all your progress?

Ah! Glad you asked…

This is where the real work comes in. Sure the detox was hard but now we need to figure out if there is a reason we want to numb out for a few minutes, a reason to not feel for just a quick minute.

This gets a little more complicated but it's really not that hard.

I was telling a coaching student yesterday that this is the time that crazy saying that no one really knows what it means comes into play:

"Listen to your body."

The trouble is you need to get past the cravings without using sugar to hear the message. The physical cravings will be lessened but…

You need to get to the emotional detox.

Talk about the stuff no one knows what it means except Ph.D. therapists…

But it's really simple.

If you believe sugar is a powerful drug, *and you will before this is over*, then you must know that consciously or unconsciously you may have been using it to cover up some negative emotions that you were starting to feel. This pattern of behavior most likely started when you were VERY, very young.

But as an adult it no longer serves you.

You need to learn the tips and tricks to walk through this reorientation of how you deal with life's everyday stressors.

It's really not that hard.

Seriously.

But as the reduced carb diet failure rate will prove it needs to be addressed if you are to succeed at this.

I think the best way to accomplish this is to decipher that old saying "listen to your body."

What you want to do is to keep asking yourself during the cravings:

"What am I really feeling?" and "what do I really need?"

It could be something as simple as a hug.

It could be a resolution to something in your relationship or your workplace. The reasons are as varied as each one of us.

Until we stop, listen and take the appropriate actions we are bound to repeat our go-to strategy of using sugar to quiet the feelings or thoughts for a minute. We learned and adopted this strategy as a very small child and it is ingrained deeply in our psyche and our brain's hard wiring. If we're to change we must change this strategy and ultimately these brain patterns.

While this sounds a little deep and not really what you signed up for please just understand this:

In working with addicts of all stripes for over thirty years one thing I do know for sure. We need to be OFF the substance before we can deal with some of these other issues.

The problem is as we detox the emotions and feelings seem to come from nowhere. The weepiness, the fear, the anxiety and more negative stuff. Even when our lives seem like they are "in a good place" - sugar withdrawals and the time period between days say 7 and 90+ are just plain weird. No other way to describe it. We go into more detail in our private groups but none of that will do you any good if you can't get through the original detox. So that's why we're here.

If you'd like to watch a video of someone actually coming to terms with a detox and committing to that you can access that right here. This is live one-on-one coaching. I'll warn you that it's a little emotional. You can watch it here

ADDICTION AND CRAVING
AND WILLPOWER, OH MY!

We at **SugarAddiction.com** believe that sugar addiction is, for some folks, a biochemical dependency that cannot be controlled by willpower alone.

Goodness knows we have all tried! Food addiction is very similar to drug addiction. Just like opiates lead to chemical addictions in the brain, ingesting flour and sugar in all its forms triggers our bodies to crave more.

Biochemical means characterized by, produced by, or involving chemical reactions in living organisms such as the brain. Those who suffer from sugar addiction experience physical cravings, mental obsession, and a distortion of basic instincts and will.

There is a lot of scientific proof related to these cravings, but since we're trying to keep this book short and sweet (if you'll pardon the pun), we're going to focus more on solutions you can implement to overcome these cravings. And, yes, you *can* overcome them!

Addiction: No One Wants To Admit To This Ugly Word

Before we move on, we need to stop and address a simple yet powerful word: **addiction**. Addiction is a tough word. It conjures up sad and very stigmatizing images of men with bottles in brown paper bags who live under bridges, overdose deaths and the opioid/heroin epidemic.

When you think of an addict, chances are you picture someone hooked on heroin or crack, needle punctures up and down their arms, living in squalor or maybe on the streets, selling anything (including their body) to get that next hit.

No one, early on, can bring themselves to relate to the idea of addiction and sugar. I seriously almost changed the name of the website because of that.

But you see I'm an addict. Today the non stigmatizing language is "a person in long term recovery from substance use disorder." I'm that too. You'll have to wait for my book on that to hear the juicy details of all that. lol

In being an addict and working with drug, alcohol and food addicts for over thirty years I come at this sugar thing a little differently than my fellow sugar educators out there.

I love them all, don't get me wrong.

They are raising the profile of sugar as a known addictive substance to previously unknown heights...

But ninety 90+ % of them are health and wellness educators. And very "in shape" type folks to boot. Not true, long term sugar addicts.

And maybe you're not a sugar addict either.

Maybe you don't want to identify as one.

I get that.

With this idea of the addict, it's easy to see why no one would want to admit to being one themselves. But addiction covers a much greater spectrum of addictive substances and behaviors.

According to the **American Society of Addiction Medicine**:

"Addiction is characterized by inability to consistently abstain, impairment in behavioral control, craving, diminished recognition of significant problems with one's behaviors and interpersonal relationships, and a dysfunctional emotional response. Like other chronic diseases, addiction often involves cycles of relapse and remission. Without treatment or engagement in recovery activities, addiction is progressive and can result in disability or premature death."

You can be addicted to food, alcohol, drugs, people, work, exercise, sex, gambling, shopping, social media—and so on. In short, addiction simply refers to a behavior over which you have no control.

The Power of Sugar and Flour

Did you know that flour turns to sugar in your stomach? That's why flour and sugar are pretty much the same when it comes to cravings. Sugar does not just contribute to weight gain; it's effects go much deeper than that.

Sugar and flour are very powerful psychoactive drugs. For some people, that wreak havoc on the body and alter how we feel and behave—in the same way that more, so called, "powerful" drugs like alcohol and cocaine do.

The problem is that people never tie together the idea of sugar and flour being "psychoactive."

They just can't seem to put them in the same category with other drugs. Even though we've all experienced the "sugar rush" or "sugar high" we still don't think of ourselves as abusers of drugs when we overeat sugar and flour.

There is plenty of research, like that done at the University of Florida, showing that certain foods, such as those that contain sugar, create the same responses in the brain's dopamine receptors as alcohol and other addictive substances. In addition, it states that sugar actually surpasses cocaine as a reward.

Intuitively, we all know that, but what kicks in is the number one symptom of addiction: denial. Who wants to admit that they are a drug addict and their drug of choice is food (or at least highly processed and refined foods)? Many recovered drug and alcohol addicts have said that it was harder to get off flour and sugar than it was to get off drugs and alcohol.

Think about that for a minute.

Does that give you an idea of just how powerful the draw is to use these substances?

Just know that it's not your fault. Flour and sugar has been in our food system long before you were even born. But armed with the information in this book, on our

website, or any other source of help, now that you're aware of the power of flour and sugar, you need to take steps to help yourself.

Cravings

A craving is a powerful desire for something. Research indicates that pretty much 100% of women and 70% of men have regular food cravings.

People who are not addicted to sugar may tell you that your cravings are all in your head, but in fact cravings are very real, biological responses. Three regions in the brain—the hippocampus, insula, and caudate—are responsible for cravings and tend to be stronger than the brain's reward center.

When you're stressed or anxious or otherwise upset, this is the moment when your craving for emotionally-satisfying foods kicks in. During your food binge your anxiety and stress seem to melt away—hence the strong "reward" factor.

Consuming flour and sugar raises serotonin, *one of our body's natural chemicals that maintains mood balance and has a calming effect.*

Volume as a Trigger

Later on in this book we will get to a healthy food plan for recovery, but please keep in mind that large volumes of food, even on the food plan, can trigger cravings. In other words, eating large amounts of food causes a change in one of the brain's chemicals, dopamine, which activates an appetite for the very food that stimulated the dopamine level in the first place.

In order to treat sugar addiction—or any addiction, actually—you must change your lifestyle. For us it means not only changing the foods that we eat but also the amount that we eat.

Check out an interview of me on The Kick Sugar Summit for a more in depth understanding of just why quitting sugar doesn't have to be hard. Our clients paid $97.00 for the interview. Yours free here. Click here!

THE MYTH OF WILLPOWER

Many people who suffer from sugar addiction (or any other form of addiction) have probably bemoaned the fact that if only they had more willpower, they could overcome their dependency on food.

Willpower is not the problem.

When it comes to sugar addiction, *nobody* has enough willpower to stop it once and for all. Roy Baumeister, a Florida State University psychologist, and New York Times science columnist John Tierney wrote a book called ***Willpower: Rediscovering the Greatest Strength*** in which they show that willpower is a form of mental energy that is fueled by glucose.

What this means is that your crumbling resolve is not a figment of your imagination or evidence that you are lazy; it means that after you deplete your glucose reserve your ability to control your actions, emotions, and choices becomes weak. Hence succumbing to temptation and making poor decisions. To quote Tierney: "We call it the dieter's catch-22: in order to not eat, you need willpower. But in order to have willpower you need to eat."

Dependency Can't Be Controlled By Willpower Alone

Since willpower is a finite resource that inevitably becomes depleted, when we put all our addiction-stopping eggs into the willpower basket, we are just setting ourselves up to fail. And no amount of willpower can make you put the carton of ice cream down if you are getting something out of it—which everyone with an addiction is.

Louise Hay distills addiction down to the belief that we're not good enough. Any type of compulsive behavior is a means of running away from all those painful, uncomfortable, and frightening feelings that are tumbling around inside of us. We binge eat to numb these feelings, and then the binge eating itself serves as a distraction from examining and dealing with the feelings.

In other words, we have a *need* to eat sugar.

It is only by acknowledging and then releasing the need that we can recover.

Abstinence

First, let us clarify exactly what we mean by abstinence. Abstinence is, in this case, a complete avoidance of sugar and flour—those substances that we constantly crave in our addiction. Avoiding these things may seem daunting, but once you begin to change your habits and experience the positive consequences as a result, you will find that abstinence gets easier.

There are two basic ways to recover from sugar addiction: incrementally or completely. In the first strategy you gradually give up trigger foods, and in the second you go cold turkey and give up all trigger foods.

The "wean off" vs cold turkey debate.

We are of the cold turkey school.

I think weaning down is a helpful process to some extent but if you want to add that to your process let's do that before the day one start date.

It will probably be a little helpful if you have a huge sugar habit to start a week out and cut down to as near zero as you can before we start cold turkey.

The goal of this whole exercise, and to some extent this entire detox, is to understand the link between your sugar use and the use of sugar as a tool for managing stress. And then to change that behavior by adding behaviors that better serve you.

We at **SugarAddiction.com** subscribe to the second model of abstinence, because we believe that giving up only some foods will still trigger cravings and cause you to either binge on another food or increase the volume of your remaining trigger foods. If you don't cut out all your addictive foods you won't be able to sustain abstinence from any of them.

We believe that when it comes to sugar addiction, moderation always fails. That's like a sober alcoholic trying to drink socially. It's a recipe for disaster.

IMPORTANT Side Note(s) here:

OK, let's take a break here. We've thrown a lot at you, you're ready to throw your e-reader, laptop or phone across the room and declare this guy nuts! I get that. I felt the same way when people told me the things above.

Let's break this down.

1. **You do not have to commit today to quitting sugar forever.**
2. Forever is a long ways off
3. All we have is today

What if you just commit to trying this little plan for one 24 hour period at a time?

Don't even think a week, a month or till your birthday. Just today. Some of the ideas and requirements of 12 step programs are not realistic for the average person - but that "Just for Today" thingy is the real deal.

Just commit to this plan for one 24 hour period. If it gets tough - just go to bed early! (Little trick I learned)

Seriously folks this is your life and your health we're talking about, maybe your kids' life and long term well-being. Hang with me and keep reading. Maybe even take a break if you have to.

WHAT TO EXPECT

Because of the catch-22 nature of cravings (sugar triggers dopamine), it is very likely that you will have to abstain from sugar and flour for the long-term.

For anyone with a dependency on a substance that provides such emotional "relief" this can seem as though you are being asked to cut off a leg. This is the reaction of the addict. But if you think about the life you desire—a happy, healthy life free from the rollercoaster of sugar addiction and binge eating and the inevitable feelings of disgust, despair, and shame—a sugar and flour-free life won't seem as scary.

I feel at this juncture I must jump in again and say this:

"Not everyone reading this book is a sugar addict. Plain and simple."

You could just have a slight dependency, you could be using sugar as a crutch. There are lots of possibilities. The honest folks who have tried over and over again they will see themselves in these pages. If that's not you then let's just trying this:

As I said, if the 12 step programs gave us one good thing it was the use and popularization of this phrase and concept: "One Day at a Time".

Why don't you, one day at a time, just try to see what life would be like sugar free?

AFTER you string together 30 or 60 days - then make your decision on whether to continue. You know you've gotten a few days or week under your belt before and lost weight and felt better.

So just try it. We are here to support any path you choose. This is a process not an instant event. If you fail the first time just regroup and try again. This journey IS worth the work.

The Benefits of Sugar and Flour Abstinence are Vast

Natural Weight Loss

Cutting out sugar and flour will automatically cause natural weight loss. Why? These foods stimulate the production of insulin, which is a hormone made by the pancreas that regulates glucose levels. Insulin controls how the body uses the fat that comes from the food we ingest, and when insulin levels are low, the body has an easier time accessing the stored fat and burning it to provide energy.

Decreased Health Risks

Abstaining from sugar and flour will lower your risk of health problems, such as diabetes, heart disease, high blood pressure, high cholesterol, and a host of other health problems listed earlier.

Improved Immune System

Eating just one teaspoon of sugar suppresses the immune system for up to five hours. A weakened immune system puts us at risk of illness including infectious diseases, allergies, and the common cold.

Self-Love

Abstinence is about more than just food; it is an emotional and spiritual journey and a means to a rich inner life of confidence, peace, and happiness.

Mental Sharpness

We all know that feeling of being in a sugar fog or sugar hangover after a binge. Your thinking is fuzzy, you feel sleepy, you become bloated, gassy, constipated, your head pounds, and your emotions swing like a monkey on a branch. Avoiding sugar and flour clears this up, making you mentally sharper and thus better able to perform daily tasks which involve thinking.

Self-Control

Sugar addiction, as we've mentioned before, is not really about the food; it's about our self-worth. Practicing abstinence will help you become more patient with yourself as you learn not to act out with food, but rather deal with whatever is really going on in that moment.

Cravings will Subside with Abstinence

Cravings occur when your body begins to detox from sugar and flour. Since you've been consuming sugar and flour for a long time, your body has built up a dependency. You will need to have a period of abstinence from sugar in order to release the compulsion to use it again.

After a week or two your cravings for sugar will begin to dissipate, and the longer you abstain the easier it will be. Just take it one day at a time and those hardcore physical cravings will no longer be part of your everyday life.

To help yourself establish a sugar-free lifestyle, it's extremely helpful (crucial, for some people) to avoid places and situations that involve sugar and flour, or any of your other trigger foods, and surround yourself with people and places that are sugar and flour-free.

For example, if you crave dessert after dinner, you may want to reach out to a friend or go for a walk after your evening meal. If you always go to the movies with friends who "have to have" sweets, try going with other friends who can support your sugar- and flour-free commitment.

Just remember that at first your cravings will cause you a lot of discomfort, then the discomfort will come and go, and finally your discomfort will diminish and eventually disappear entirely. It's only normal for addicts to want to feel great immediately, but unfortunately that's not how it works. Remember, it took years for your body and your mind to become addicted to sugar, so it will take some time to reverse this addiction.

A Bonus Side Note and a Vision of the Future about the Growling Stomach

When I was a kid and I "thought" I was hungry my stomach would growl. Now I'm not talking about a little grumbling noise here. I talking about a real growling sound that could be heard by others across a table! You know that ache in your stomach like it's empty and it adds strange sounds to it? ...Yes, that feeling.

Well here's the take away: What I've come to know is a growling stomach is not hunger! It's sugar and flour withdrawals. Yes for the last over 25 years my stomach hasn't growled. No noises at all when I'm hungry. Try it for yourself.

The Importance of Beginning, Nurturing, Guarding, and Loving Abstinence

We cannot emphasize enough how important it is to learn to love your abstinence. Not just *be* abstinent, but truly love it. Just because you have been able to successfully stop eating sugar does not necessarily mean that your binging days are over.

If you're abstaining from sugar and flour but quietly (or not so quietly) resenting the fact that you "have to," your risk of relapse will always be right around the corner. And, as the previous section on cravings showed, one relapse can trigger a nose-dive right back into your sugar addiction.

But if you are willing to begin your abstinence, nurture it like it's a newborn baby, guard it with the same determination that you hid your use of sugar, and love it with everything you've got, then you will find that your chance of relapsing is greatly decreased. So long as you are serious about, and seriously in love with, abstaining from sugar and flour, happiness will be your lifelong companion.

One of THE most watched and commented on videos in our library is "The Myth of Willpower" video. If you'd like to check it out here we've set up a free copy of it for you.

WITHDRAWALS

Many books on how to stop eating sugar, and even, sadly, some counselors, seem to pay little attention to the process of withdrawal. Once you cut out sugar and flour (or any addictive substance), your physical and emotional attachment to them is not going to disappear overnight. The body goes through a period of detoxification as it rids the system of every last trace of these toxic substances.

But once you get over the initial hump through abstinence, you will begin to feel so much better and you will be on your way to having your use under control.

Sugar addiction will no longer control you.

What to Expect with Withdrawals

If you've ever tried to stop eating sugar, you know the consequences you go through, from headaches to cold-like symptoms. Those effects are indicative of just how powerful sugar is on your system, both physically and emotionally.

Sugar and flour withdrawal symptoms include:

- hunger (this is not real hunger, it's emotional hunger)
- headache
- faster heartbeat
- lethargy, low energy, tired all the time
- mood swings
- anger
- anxiety, depression,
- sadness or grief over the loss of this substance
- digestive problems such as diarrhea or cramps
- insomnia

- cold or flu-like symptoms such as chills, sweating, runny nose, watery eyes
- Anxiety is heightened
- You may feel weepy and very emotional for a time

Depending on various factors—such as how long you've been eating sugar and flour and your personal health—these withdrawal symptoms could last a few weeks or a few months, but as long as you stick with it, eventually the withdrawal symptoms go away—along with your craving for foods with flour or sugar.

If natural weight loss is a benefit of cutting out sugar and flour, then why can't we just wake up one day and say: "That's it! For thirty days I will eat no flour and no sugar!"—and then keep our promise to ourselves?

In most aspects of our lives we function and perform tasks that we don't love but we do anyway because we're adults and we know they're our responsibility. But

when it comes to not using flour and sugar it's obvious by the growing obesity epidemic that we aren't able to say we are going to quit and then actually do it.

Why is that?

Most people can't do that simple exercise because of cravings. What are sugar cravings? Simple. Sugar withdrawals. It's your body wanting to re-ingest its poison.

The first day you go off sugar and flour the cravings aren't too bad. But if you are like most people, within two or three days you will be a basket case. (Yes, that is a medical term!) You will literally not be able to function well. You'll likely experience

all manner of the withdrawal symptoms listed above. In short, you will not be fun to be around.

I know this is going to scare some people off and I'm okay with that. You'll be back when you're ready.

How to Cope with Withdrawals

The answer to that million-dollar question "So how do I stop sugar cravings?" is abstinence.

You need to have a period of abstinence from sugar and flour in order for the compulsion to use it again to be released. Words like "compulsion" might be difficult to accept at first, but if you're reading this book then you're clearly ready and open-minded enough to face it.

You need to string together a week or more of sugar- and flour-free living in order to allow the sugar cravings to dissipate. Keep in mind that it will take much longer than a week to overcome the urge to use sugar all together, but the hardcore physical cravings will not be a part of your everyday life if you can commit to this initial period of abstinence.

We have found that people need to do two things to get through this initial detox, as well as the first few months of abstinence, and go on to a happier, healthier, and (as a result) thinner life.

1. You Need Information

With all the confusing and often conflicting information out there, you need to be able to separate fact from fiction. Addiction and health are two of the most confusing topics out there for the average person. As we stated at the beginning of this book, we take sugar addiction very seriously and strive to provide the very best information and support for this disorder that is causing immense pain worldwide, and to help people like you to gain control over your sugar and thus your life. We've been there ourselves, so we know exactly how you feel.

2. You Need Support

In order to beat an addiction or issue that has plagued you for years, you cannot do it alone. Support groups are often looked upon as havens for weak people who can't do it themselves, can't "pull themselves up by their bootstraps," and can't "just stop" like all the people around them are telling them to do.

But the evidence of success for people helping others do anything is well documented throughout history. We humans are a social bunch. We need each other and we act and react better when we are in a group setting.

One of the biggest common denominators among people who are successful—at anything, not just stopping binge eating—is that they never did it alone. They always had support, whether it was a mentor, a friend, a therapist, a 12-step program, or any other form of assistance and encouragement. (More on this later.)

Remember, your attachment to sugar and flour is emotional and won't disappear after one day of abstinence. Please be patient with and kind to yourself, and enlist whichever type of support works best for you.

Day-by-day Outline of Walking Through and Managing Withdrawal

If you're 100% ready, willing, and open, I'm going to walk you through sugar and flour withdrawal (and make no mistake—that is exactly what it is). The hardest part will be that first week or ten days.

A quick note about caffeine before we get started. Anything with caffeine in it is just going to trigger you. About 99% of caffeinated products also have sugar in it (or used with it). So I would suggest that you take one week to quit caffeine before you attempt quitting flour and sugar.

If you attempt it while going through flour and sugar withdrawal, you're going to confuse the detox symptoms and withdrawal symptoms of sugar with the detox symptoms and withdrawal symptoms of caffeine and be unable to identify each for the future. Plus the resulting physical condition of doing both at the same time is just too hard.

I also want to mention that I've seen people quit sugar and continue caffeine and it always turns out badly. They substituted large amounts of caffeine for the missing sugar buzz and then had anxiety issues. Caffeine may be right up there with nicotine in how hard it is to quit so driving your addiction to that deeper is just not wise. Without the ability to use sugar at night to "take the edge off" a day of caffeine use (A) you might never get any sleep and (B) the anxiety is overwhelming.

Work schedule: I always suggest that if you can't take a week off during this withdrawal process then start on a Friday. The first day of going off sugar and flour won't be so bad, and then you'll have the weekend.

Family: You will need to prepare them because you're not going to be yourself. Try to plan this for a time when your obligations in general are at their lowest. We want you to be able to rest a lot.

Food preparation: Be prepared!! Throw out absolutely everything with sugar and flour in it. Have the foods you *can* eat on hand, and have lots of them. While I do believe that some people are triggered by volume of food, eating a little more of non-sugar and flour items during withdrawals is fine.

Make this your priority: The most important thing to do, one day at a time, is not ingest flour or sugar. Take short walks every day and rest. A lot. Your body needs it—badly. Your adrenals and other feel good glands are beat to hell and need a rest. During that rest they are not functioning that well so as a result you feel bad physically.

WIllpower: Or should I say "The Myth of Willpower." Willpower does not work. Period, end of story. We have one of our most popular videos for you right here, aptly named: "The Myth of Willpower" yours to watch for FREE.

Detox Outline/Timeline

Now we will walk you through exactly what is going to happen and exactly what you should do every day as you transition off sugar.

When we start we will be talking about zero sugar consumption daily. At least for a time period of your choosing.

Day 1: Grace Day. It's a strange phenomena really. For some with super heavy habits the end of the day gets rough but usually the body is just so happy not to have to process out the toxin that you feel pretty OK. A little tired and a possible headache near the end of the day but manageable.

To do: Be prepared for the next day food wise and schedule wise. Make this your priority. This is the day you change your life. Make it special.

Day 2: The going gets a little rougher. Hopefully you've followed the instructions above and have the day to rest. Eat your three solid meals. No snacking in between.

Now you are going to start feeling headaches, possibly severe ones. These can start today or any day up to and past even day four.

I would implore you NOT to use any pain medication. Please. We are trying to go in the other direction.

Would it shock you to know I haven't had a headache in over thirty years? On the other side awaits a life free of headaches.

You're also going to be tired and depressed. Take heart it's not a mental issue. It's just your brain adjusting to not having the physical manipulations of the sugar and down regulating your feel good brain chemicals to begin the healing process.

Remember you will feel all of this and more:

- You will be emotional.

- You may be inexplicably weepy.

- You'll be angry for no reason.

- Sad for no reason.

- You'll be a little depressed. Not to worry it's not a mental issue it's a physical withdrawal symptom.

- The stress will feel unbearable at times.

Take a nap. Possibly the first one in your adult life? But DO IT. Take a short walk. Twenty minutes. Go to yoga or the gym. Any of these will help you sleep(nap and at night).

Symptom Alert!

Now here's a tough one: You are going to feel like you are STARVING. Possibly for days. You obviously are not.

Some people have a tough time with overeating and then not being able to control that even after they are sugar-free. But I would suggest that you can eat as much as you like of anything on the food plan below and go heavy on the good fats to get through this starving feeling.

It will pass, as will all the withdrawals.

To do: Nap, walk, lots of water. Journal in a cheap separate notebook how you felt. Remember it and be able to look back at it when you feel like using some sugar - would you want to go through that again?

Journaling your feelings is important. Very much in the early days but also as you get more time and heal up and the "cravings" start again.

Day 3: Read Day Two above again… sorry to be the bearer of bad news.

Quick side note. Somewhere between days one and five you may have the night sweats. This is perfectly normal. Please no running to the doctor for some kind of medicine. It is a sugar withdrawal symptom. One, by the way, you may be having now. Then, in some people, if they get sugar after being sugar free. This is a dead giveaway that your body is quickly trying to detox it.

Day 4: There may be a little break in the "awfulness". Depending on your sugar habit going in. A lot of people are through the worst of it in a few days. Some, sadly, are in for a few more days of the same as day two above. (Groundhog Day)

No matter which you are, you're gonna be OK.

You may be back at work so there will be additional challenges. The main goal is emotional management. Steer clear of emotional entanglements the best you can for a few more days.

Now it goes without saying that you are eating the right foods, in the right amount and at the right times throughout this entire detox…

- but as I said we will be focused on your emotional well being mostly.

Day 5: The Clouds Start to Clear a Little Some of Us…

If you start to feel a little better physically then your habit is a manageable one and you should walk right out of this. Your physical dependence is not that huge. If you're still on day two above then your habit was a big one and/or your body is super sensitive. In either case I would suggest continuing the things we know work. Lots of rest, as much as you can, avoid stress, lots of water, walk at least 20 minutes a day and of course stick to your sugar free diet.

Day 6: Some of us may be entering the Pink Cloud Phase…

What the heck, you ask, is a "Pink Cloud?"

A pink cloud is a feeling of euphoria. A feeling so good it tricks you into feeling like "you got this handled" or "that was easy". Please, please do NOT fall into this trap.

The pink cloud can come anytime between days 5 and 10 or even after for folks with heavy habits.

The body is physically detoxed from sugar. You're rested, hydrated and well fed. You've done a little exercise and well, hell, you just feel great.

Danger - Will Robinson - Danger! I'm dating myself. It was a TV show, Lost in Space, when I was growing up about a family trapped in space and the family robot would warn the cute son of danger.

This is precisely where people fail. (The first time)

We figure "aw heck that was easy!" I can use a little sugar… WRONG.

If I had a nickel for every time I've seen this…

We start to feel better and abandon our plan. We make up our own plan and that plan includes "just a little sugar."

Please know that your journey to wellness is just beginning. Enjoy the heck out of the pink cloud but always remember that:

- **if you use sugar you will have to repeat the last five days.**

So many people get to the point after just a few tries at detoxing that they just can't physically do it again.

They say things like "I don't have another detox in me." And then they just resign themselves to a life of health and weight issues.

Don't be that person.

Just relax and get ready for the pink cloud to end.

Week 2: During the second week, you'll start to feel better physical rather quickly. You'll start to think, "I got this." While confidence is good, overconfidence is deadly. Stick with the food plan. Begin to measure your portions and start to get in a rhythm with your schedule.

Weeks 3 and 4: Physically you'll feel much better, but many folks have a tough time emotionally. Stick to your food plan and start working on building your support system. You are going feel overwhelmed. Please don't use these feelings as an excuse to find another substitute for chemically managing your emotions.

The third and fourth weeks are very, very important because while the main physical withdrawal symptoms are gone, the re-learning of emotional sobriety is ever present. These weeks will be modeling your life moving forward.

Emotional recovery: By week two, if not earlier, you are going notice feelings of all kinds that just seem to be overwhelming you. And they all are going feel like they are hitting you at once.

This is a critical time for you and your recovery.

I personally believe that sugar and flour are not foods at all but very powerful psychoactive drugs.

Where I see the biggest failure rate is the inability to accept the idea that we have been using flour and sugar to manage our emotions our whole lives and that without it we need to learn new methods.

Your life will continue. Your stressors will continue. All your relationships will continue. What won't continue is your go-to stress reliever and your go-to escape method.

We need to find new ways to deal with the ups and downs of life. As you'll see in the exercise section, exercise is not for weight loss, it's a positive method to deal with stress.

Somewhere between days seven and twenty one, it's different for everyone depending on the severity of their habit, you are going to start feeling better physically. See "pink cloud" above.

Now is where the real work starts…

Before we dive into all that let me tell you a story about "retreads." in our practice.

Retreads are the people who "keep coming back." They get to different places of abstinence from or very low intake of sugar and then they fall off the wagon. Not only do they fall off the wagon but the wheels fall off said wagon too. It's a mess, they're a mess.

Sadly, for some of us - me included, it just seems to be part of the process.

We just get back to work with them. No judgement, no shame. So if that happens to you during the process just log back into the daily detox group, see you're not alone, fess-up and get back to it!

Maybe you've experienced this before?

In the "non addict" world they call this yo-yo dieting.

The really sad part is that we here at SugarAddiction.com have the answer to this worldwide phenomena.

You see Yo-yo dieting is just a sugar relapse.

It's an emotional relapse - not a physical one.

It's getting through the first week, month or longer, losing a little weight and then (and no-one, previous to joining us, could understand WHY) they go back to their old ways.

Quotes like: "Then I was just eating dessert" or "I don't even know how it got in my mouth."

Followed by: "I went on a week long run and ate all the things I had missed." or "I stayed away from the things I was successful with and gained back all the weight I lost plus ten extra pounds!"

Hundreds of times this has happened.

Getting to the DEEP understanding of ourselves as to why this happens is the true key to success with quitting or controlling sugar in our lives - not what we eat or how many sit-ups we do.

It's giving sugar the respect it deserves as a mood and mind altering drug and then using the experience and success of hundreds of thousands of people, who have had success with addictions large and small, to succeed ourselves in controlling sugar in our lives.

So let's return to days 7 to 14, depending on your habit, through day 30 and beyond.

I want you to focus now on **"the emotional detox."**

After the sugar is out of our system we will have some relief from the strong physical cravings that have always derailed us before.

With support from the Facebook group you won't feel as alone and, to be honest, you'll feel a little braver about taking this to the next level.

The next level, as I've hinted at above, is really the rewiring and reconfiguring of our brain and emotions to handle everyday stress.

The danger zones in this second phase of your recovery, your long term recovery, are all mental and emotional. When you succeed with the physical elimination of sugar from your body you are prepared to tackle what really keeps you in control.

This is a hard topic for some people - I get that.

First it takes a long time to just accept that sugar has had such a strong effect on our feelings and emotions. That little girl you once were who soothed her upset (and whose mother did too) with candy and cookies is still using the same methods as an adult. The really difficult part for folks to accept is the power of sugar to do such a thing to our brain, our emotions and our psyche.

The idea that this universally accepted sweet, that we give to children is being maligned, slandered! This I would say is one of the hardest leaps we need to make.

If you're in the Facebook group already or followed our public Facebook group then I'm preaching to the choir. That's good. But for you folks that need just a little more convincing then I ask you this: If I told you no steak, or your favorite veggie if you're vegetarian, for say six months how would you feel?

Well maybe you'd be bummed a little but there are plenty of other options and as an adult you could handle it.

What if I also told you that if you did your weight would fall to it's normal body weight for you, you might be able to get off all your diabetes meds, your skin would look better, you'd sleeping better, you'd have more motivation etc… You'd probably do it.

Well now ponder this:

You've know in your heart that quitting or controlling sugar in your life would do all these things. You tried many times before. But for some reason all those "it's the diet, the food and the exercise" folks have not been able to help you to sustain long term.

So why is it so hard?

It's hard because it takes four legs to a stool to complete this task 100%.

Here they are:

1. Sugar Abstinence and Food
2. Family and Environment
3. Mind and Emotions
4. Self Care and Peer Support

If you fall short on any of these four then your stool falls over.

1. Eat ANY sugar and we end up fighting the - physical cravings.
2. A toxic home or workplace filled with sugar and pressure? = Binge.
3. Not prepared mentally and ignoring how you feel emotionally = relapse.
4. All alone in this and not caring for yourself = the easiest way to fail!

The concepts of the four basics above are the basis of a solid long term success with sugar.

Some are tricky, some are nuanced. It takes the support of people who have walked this way before to walk through it.

While this small book was designed to GET you off sugar, our private group was created to KEEP you off sugar and to help if you fall back.

Theoretically you could do any of the popular detoxes out there and we encourage folks to try different ways to get through the initial physical detox. The question you then have ask is: What then?

Failure means going through the pain of detox a second or third time. Sometimes even more than three.

Why not join us in the private group now and just do this once? LINK

Get all four legs of your stool in place as you move through the first phase of the physical.

Because - you do know the the mental and emotional issues start right away right? They are just overshadowed by the physical.

It's just a joy to work with people who are serious about regaining their health and vitality.

We will see you on the inside of The Daily Sugar Detox Group. Click here to get access to the group and more bonuses

Just to calm your nerves, about thinking about the future of your life with or without sugar, I got permission from my client to let you watch an one of my entire hour long coaching sessions. In it you'll see how gentle the process described below is in real life. This particular person is coming up on a year sugar free by doing exactly what you're doing here. Check it out here

FOOD PLAN FOR RECOVERY

An essential part of your recovery from sugar addiction is having a solid, healthy food plan in place as you eliminate sugar and flour from your diet. The foundation of the food plan is the most important step in obtaining abstinence, and it is imperative that we follow our plan for the amounts we eat and how often, which we will get to in a bit.

Eating healthy foods and cutting out toxic ones affects the mind in a positive way, meaning that sound nutritional habits will aid you in gaining control over the insanity of this dependency.

Once you begin following the plan you may be tempted to deviate—even just a teensy bit—or give yourself a "well-deserved" cheat day. Please keep in mind that the tendency to rationalize is part of an addict's thinking, so you'll need to summon up a little extra strength and courage to win over these temptations, and trust that these are proven guidelines that have helped countless others who have been there just like you. It worked for us, and it will work for you.

Benefits of Following the Food Plan

You're going to see a lot of food in the coming pages, so please keep in mind that, even if you're on the food plan, these foods can trigger cravings as well. The food plan is not a diet; dieting doesn't help sugar addiction. In order to treat sugar addiction—any addiction, actually—you must change your lifestyle.

For us it means changing the foods that we eat, the way that we eat them, and the amount that we eat. The guidelines for men, women and children vary, so there is no one, across-the-board plan for everyone to follow.

These are just some of the benefits you'll discover when you follow the food plan:

- Develop healthy eating habits
- Reduce/eliminate cravings for sugar, flour
- Clear the body and mind of chemicals that inhibit healthy and positive thinking

- Heal our internal organs that may have been damaged by binge eating abuse
- Enable our bodies to operate at optimal levels
- Stabilize blood sugar levels and metabolism to prevent triggering cravings and binges
- Gain self-confidence, which lowers our desire to sabotage ourselves

NSFW: No Sugar, Flour & Wheat

Ok, you now know that you need to abstain from sugar and flour but what does that mean exactly?

SUGAR - Do you have any idea how many different types of sugar there are? Check out this list (in alphabetical order):

- Ace-K
- Acesulfame-k (Sunette, Sweet and Safe, Sweet One)
- Aguamiel
- Alcohol
- Alitame
- Amasake

- Artificial Sweeteners such as Equal, Sweet 'n Low, Splenda, etc. (Please note: All diet sodas have artificial sweeteners, which are now known to create cravings similar to sugar.)

- Artificial flavors (some)
- Aspartame/Nutrasweet
- Barley malt
- Cane juice/Evaporated cane juice
- Caramel coloring
- Concentrated fruit juice
- Corn sweetener
- Cyclamates
- Date paste/syrup
- Dextrin
- Dried/dehydrated fruit
- Extracts
- Fat substitutes made from concentrated fruit paste
- Fructooligosaccharides (FOS)
- Fruit flavorings (some)
- Glucosamine/glucosamine
- Glycerine
- Honey
- Jaggery
- Licorice root powder
- Light, lite or low sugar products
- Malted barley
- Maltodextrins

- Malts
- Molasses/blackstrap molasses
- "Natural" flavors (some)
- "Natural" sweeteners
- Nectars
- Neotame
- Olestra (made from sucrose)
- Raisin juice, paste or syrup
- Rice malt, sugar or syrup
- Rice sweeteners
- Saccharin

- Sorghum
- Stevia
- Sucanat (evaporated cane juice)
- Sucraryl
- Sugars: apple sugar, Barbados sugar, bark sugar, beet sugar, brown sugar, cane sugar, caramel sugars, confectioner's sugar, date sugar, grape sugar, invert sugar, milled sugar, "natural" sugar, powdered sugar, raw sugar, turbinado sugar, unrefined sugar, etc.
- Syrups: agave, barley, brown rice, corn, date, high-fructose corn, maple, raising, yinnie (rice), etc.
- Vanillin
- Whey (as an additive)
- Xanthan gum

And anything with the following suffixes contains sugar:

- **-ides:** monosodium glycerides, polyglycerides, disaccharides, trisaccharides, diglycerides, disaccharides, glycerides, monoglycerides, monosaccharides, etc.
- **-ol:** carbitol, glucitol, glycol, hexitol, inversol, maltitol, mannitol, sorbitol, xylitol, etc.
- **-ose:** colorose, dextrose, fructose, galactose, glucose, lactose, levulose, mannose, polydextrose, polytose, ribose, sucralose, sucrose, tagatose, zylose

FLOUR - As you might recall, flour turns to sugar in your stomach.

- Beans, vegetables, nuts or grains that are ground into flour, meal or powder
- Guar gum
- Starches

WHEAT

- Bran (if made from wheat)
- Bulgar
- Cracked wheat
- Durum wheat

- Gluten
- Kamut

- Red wheat/red spring wheat
- Seitan (made from wheat protein, gluten)
- Semolina
- Spelt
- Triticale (a wheat/rye hybrid)
- Wheat berries
- Wheat flakes
- Wheat germ
- Whole-grain wheat
- Winter wheat

It's a really good idea to get into the habit of checking labels for lists of ingredients, as you may find other names for sugar, flour, and wheat. Please be aware that some products contain sugar naturally, so make sure you're checking the ingredients list and not the nutrition facts, which will list sugars naturally contained in such ingredients as fruits and vegetables. The more informed you are about what you need to avoid, the easier it will be to know what to look for.

Food Plan: How Much and How Often

This food plan is a guide. Notice we said "guide," not magic wand. Please keep in mind that anyone jumping in and following a food plan when they are not also immersed in the inner work such as therapy, 12-steps, or other support groups like our private Facebook group will likely find that the food plan will only be a temporary measure. It's difficult implementing a new lifestyle (such as a new way of eating) without support and resources and like-minded people with whom to share your struggles.

Breakfast	Lunch (4 hours later)	Dinner (5 hours later)	Snack (4 hours later)
1 protein	1 protein	1 protein	1 dairy or 2 oz. protein
1 dairy	1 cooked vegetable	1 cooked vegetable	1 fruit

1 fruit	1 fresh vegetable	1 fresh vegetable
1 grain or starchy vegetable	½ daily oil	1 grain or starchy vegetable
	Men: add 1 fruit or 1 grain or 1 starchy vegetable	½ daily oil

Getting your sugar addiction under control and being on the road to recovery is about *all* foods and beverages. Here we provide a list of appropriate protein, vegetable, starch, dairy, condiment, fat, grain and beverage choices.

PROTEIN

Beef	4 oz.
Chicken	4 oz.
Dried beans	1 c. cooked
Eggs	2 medium
Fish	4 oz.
Hot dogs (not sugar cured)	4 oz.
Lamb	4 oz.
Pork	4 oz.
Shellfish	4 oz.
Turkey	4 oz.
Veal	4 oz.
Vegetarian protein (tofu, tempeh)	6 oz.

VEGETABLES (1 cup of any of the following)

artichoke	mushroom	Brussels sprouts	romaine	cucumber	tomatoes
asparagus	okra	cabbage	rutabaga	dill pickles	turnips
bamboo shoots	onions	carrots	sauerkraut	eggplant	vegetable juice

beans (yellow or green)	peppers	cauliflower	snow pea pods	endive
bok choy	pimentos	celery	spinach	escarole
beets	radishes	chicory	summer squash	greens *
broccoli	rhubarb	Chinese cabbage	Swiss chard	watercress

*** beet, collard, dandelion, kale, all types of lettuce, mustard, any sprouts (no wheat grass)

Note – tomato juice or vegetable cocktail juice without sugar may be used as a cooked vegetable substitute. 1 cup juice =1 cup cooked vegetables.

FRUITS

Apple	1 medium
Applesauce	1/2 c.
Apricots	3 medium
Berries	1 c.
Cantaloupe	1/2 (6" dia.)
Cherries	1 c.
Grapefruit	1/2 large
Grapes	1 c.
Honeydew	1/4 (7" dia.)
Kiwi	3 small
Lemons, limes	2 small/ 1 large
Nectarines	2 small/ 1 large
Orange	1 large
Peach	1 large
Pear	1 large
Pineapple	1 c.

Plums	3 med.
Tangerine	2 small

STARCHES

Baked potato (white)	1 small (6 oz.)
Beans (lima, navy, all dried beans)	1/2 c. cooked
Corn	1 med.

Corn (kernel)	1/2 c. cooked
Mashed potatoes (white)	1/2 c.
Mashed yams	1/2 c.
Parsnips	1/2 c.
Peas, dried	1/2 c.
Peas, green	1/2 c.
Pumpkin	1/2 c.
Sweet potato	1 small (6 oz.)
Squash*	1/2 c.

***acorn, butternut, Hubbard, winter and spaghetti squash*

DAIRY

Buttermilk	1 c.
Ricotta cheese	1/2 c.
Milk	1 c.
Cottage cheese	1/2 c.
Plain yogurt	1 c.
Unsweetened soy beverage	1 c.

****Note – if you are dairy sensitive, eliminate dairy and substitute 2 oz. of any type of protein.*

*We would suggest that if you can do without dairy to do so. Many, many of our clients have trouble until they remove dairy as well. But that can come after you are stable and totally free of all processed sugar and flour if you like. ****

CONDIMENTS - Any spice or sauce that is sugar-free, alcohol-free or wheat-free including, but not limited to, mustard, tamari, salsa, non-fat yogurt, lemon juice, etc. Limit spice and condiment use to the levels recommended in recipes or no more than 1 teaspoon per day of any one spice and no more than two tablespoons per day of any one sauce.

FAT (Women choose one and men choose two from the following)

Oil (olive, coconut)	1 tablespoon
Butter	1 tablespoon
Mayonnaise - sugar free	1 tablespoon
Salad dressing (without sugar, artificial sweetener, or corn syrup)	2 tablespoons

Grains (1 cup of any of the following, measured after cooking)

Amaranth	Grits
Barley	Millet
Brown rice	Oat bran*
Buckwheat	Oatmeal
	Quinoa

***(1/2 c. raw=1 c. cooked) + Non-wheat, sugar-free, dry cereal*

The same caution as with the dairy above. Many people simply can not use anything in this grain category and be successful. Only you know your body. Many folks could transition to grain and dairy free after but many had to eliminate them right from the start. In our advanced coaching most people go grain and dairy free. *

BEVERAGES - Suggested drinks are water, carbonated water, herbal tea, decaffeinated coffee or decaffeinated tea.

Clear soup (without sugar) is permitted before lunch or dinner.

Vegetable cocktail juice without sugar may be used as a cooked vegetable substitute. 1 cup juice =1 cup cooked vegetables.

Please note: All diet sodas have artificial sweeteners, which are now known to create cravings similar to sugar. Even the "flavored waters" with "natural ingredients" - please steer clear of them.

A few more words about the food plan. You're going to have questions. Ask them on the forum. Don't just guess.

A couple simple rules though. Eat just meals. For now, your life of "snacking" all the time needs to be put on hold. Self-honesty and self-examination during this process yields so much more than a thin body. It yields peace of mind and a true and deep belief in yourself and your ability to have control of your own destiny.

What would that be worth to you?

JOURNALING: A TOOL FOR SUCCESS

Journaling is a great tool for success from sugar addiction or any other type of addiction or compulsion, because it enables us to shine a light on our deepest, darkest thoughts. Shame hides in the darkness, so when we throw that floodlight on it, it has nowhere to go. It cannot have the same hold on us when it has been exposed.

Journaling is like therapy, only instead of telling someone else, you're telling yourself via a notebook. It allows you to take those sometimes cryptic or nebulous thoughts and focus them into concrete words. Journaling is also an effective way to track your progress, motivate and inspire you, and possibly even reduce your chances of relapse.

Further benefits of journaling include: clarity, learning more about yourself, gaining insight about what's going on, an outlet for stress, increasing accountability, and reminding yourself how far you've come.

The Importance of Rigorous Honesty

Here's the key, though. The difference between successful people and the ones who fail is that the people who were able to stay off sugar didn't only record what they ate, they recorded how they *felt* when they ate it.

I would like to encourage you to do the same. If you're honest in your journaling, you will start to see a very distinct pattern in your feelings and in your use of sugar. My successful clients always start to find out things like:

"Felt down and anxious before three slices of cake, but after and during—just for a few minutes—I felt right with the world. Then I crashed again and it was even worse."

"Ate 8 oz broiled salmon and 8 oz broccoli, felt the same before and after."

"I can't believe I ate a one pound bag of M&Ms, but the stress of work melted away."

"The cravings for chocolate don't seem to hit me on the weekends."

And so on and so forth.

This is a simple system, requiring just a 99¢ notebook, but it has changed many lives for the better. There is no need to change your eating patterns just yet; simply record your food intake *honestly*.

Remember to record not just your food, but also your feelings. Three easy questions:

1. How did you feel before binging or having "just a little sugar"?
2. What did your mind tell you about what you were eating and why you were eating it?
3. How did you feel afterwards?

Journal like this for one month and then review it. I think you will find that, without a shadow of a doubt, you use food (and particularly sugar) to manage your emotions, if only for a few brief moments.

This task requires that you be very honest with yourself. Remember that no one but you ever needs to read what you wrote, so if you find yourself being anything less than honest in your notebook, ask yourself who you are trying to fool.

The people who succeed, stay close to sugar free, and reach their goal weight are rigorously honest in this process of uncovering their feelings around the use of this

drug. Remember, there is no need to change your eating patterns just yet. We have to change the way that we think about sugar, and the change in diet will just happen—almost like magic.

BODY IMAGE

Recovering will be much easier if you can learn to accept your body at every stage of the process. Your journey will not only be easier, but more pleasant, too, if you surround yourself with people who are traveling the same path. Just the sheer act of talking to a like-minded fellow on the phone or meeting them for lunch will provide relief, even if only for that moment, from your thoughts of shame or self-criticism of your body.

Acceptance at All Weights

This is so much easier said than done, especially with the media bombarding us with societal expectations of what we should look like in order to be okay/lovable/accepted. Most of these images we see are, for the most part, unattainable.

This is not just an external problem; our internal thoughts about our bodies are often our worst enemy. Even people who are considered physically attractive can suffer from negative body image. There are a lot of emotional components to how we feel about our bodies and those emotions can be triggered by external forces.

Here are some external forces that can cause negative body image:

- Being bullied and/or teased as a child or mistreated as an adult
- Loneliness
- Experiencing prejudice or discrimination because of your weight, body size or lifestyle
- Being shamed by others
- Being stared at or teased for your weight (whether too heavy or too thin)
- Getting bypassed for a promotion and/or raise because of your weight
- Media and societal pressure regarding obesity and placing too much value on being thin

Part of the recovery process, and what we will help you with, is learning to love the body you are in, *no matter what size or shape you are*. We are all beautiful beings and we are all okay/lovable/acceptable just as we are.

We realize that learning to love the body we have is easier said than done and it does take practice, so that is why we encourage you to join others who are on the same journey.

Self-acceptance can sometimes be hard when we feel we've abused our body with food or sugar. We've prepared a great video with affirmations on being kind to yourself. No charge, just an adjunct to the book to help you walk through all this with dignity. Watch it here

SELF-CARE AND EXERCISE: WORKING OUT AND WORKING WITHIN

Practicing self-care is the antidote to negative self-talk, poor body image, and inability to take action (or taking the "wrong" action). It is such a simple concept that it can be easy to overlook it.

While you are fighting the good fight to overcome sugar and flour cravings, it is imperative that you balance your work with a little play, a.k.a. self-care. Since the effects of this disorder tend to be in the realm of self-loathing, being kind to yourself—even if it seems frivolous—is an important part of the plan. And bear this in mind: what might feel like a frivolity to you is usually a necessity to someone else, so perhaps a change in your perspective about yourself is in order.

There are a lot of different ways you can take care of yourself and some of them may surprise you, but, trust us, they really work.

So this is where I tell you to go get a massage.

Your entire being is saying: I don't need a massage, I need to lose X amount of weight, or I need to stop eating sugar!

I hear you.

Now go get that massage.

Self-care is defined, quite simply, as being kind to yourself. You do this mostly with self-talk but also, as I'm about to show you, in performing little acts of kindness that you have been putting off or that you've been doing for others instead of yourself.

Examples of Self-Care

- Treat yourself to a massage
- Get a mani-pedi
- Buy yourself an affordable gift, something that makes you smile
- Spend an afternoon with the kids in the pool
- Unplug from your phone and computer and relax with a new book
- Do a kind deed for someone else
- Volunteer at a local charity
- Take your neighbor's dog for a walk
- Take a walk on the beach with a friend you haven't seen in a long time
- Join a dance class
- Learn how to play an instrument
- Take an art class
- Spend the afternoon at a museum

- Join a gym and set attainable goals for yourself to get in shape (works physically and mentally)
- Tackle a project you've been putting off, such as organizing a closet, cleaning out the garage, or donating old clothes to Goodwill

If you can spend just 50% of the day saying kind things like "It's been a good day, I've stayed on my food plan and I went in the pool with the kids" instead of "I'm such a loser, I'll never be able to quit sugar," then you are well on your way to recovering.

EXERCISE: IT'S NOT WHAT YOU THINK

Exercise is for managing your emotions first, not for physical health and certainly not for weight loss.

What the heck does *that* mean?

Exercise is the "make me feel good" replacement for sugar and flour.

Obviously, a by-product of exercise is weight loss, but it's important to stop the sugar first, and understanding the role that exercise really plays in stopping it is key.

Exercise doesn't just affect the body, it affects your mental and emotional state, too. Regular exercise can relieve stress, decrease depression and anxiety, improve your sleep, and boost your mood.

We want you to think about exercise in terms of healing your adrenal glands, your serotonin uptake processes, and all the ways the body feels good naturally. After years of abuse and artificial activation, these mechanisms are simply beat to hell. They can't function as God or nature intended.

How Exercise Helps in Recovering From Sugar Addiction

Exercise will heal these mechanisms, albeit slowly. The key here is, as the Nike slogan goes, "Just do it." Just let go of the idea of burning calories or losing weight for now. What you want to do is heal the parts of your body that keep forcing you to use the substances you know you need to quit. This is a mental game mostly and you need all of your natural feel goods working.

Here's how regular exercise can help you:

- **Boosts your mood** – Exercise releases endorphins, which are a group of hormones in your brain that give you energy and make you feel good. As well as helping to relieve depression and anxiety, regular exercise may also help prevent you from relapsing.
- **Increases self-esteem** – Regular activity is something you do for yourself, so it can positively affect your sense of self-worth as you feel a sense of achievement.
- **Improves sleep** – It doesn't take much exercise to start improving your sleep. If you exercise at night, choose moderate, stretching exercises such as walking or yoga.
- **Increases energy** – To give yourself a boost of energy, start your morning off with even a few minutes of exercise. Daily exercise also strengthens your immune system.
- **Allows you to cope better** – Exercise is helpful in dealing with life's stresses in a healthy way, instead of resorting to binge eating (or any other addiction), which makes you feel worse.

How to Create a Realistic Exercise Plan

To enjoy the benefits of exercise, you don't need to turn into Dwayne "The Rock" Johnson. Just 30 minutes of moderate exercise five times a week ought to do it, or even breaking it down into two 15-minute or three 10-minute exercise sessions will do. The point is to do something and do it regularly.

If you're new to exercise or it's been a while, start with 5- or 10-minute period and then slowly increase your time. It may feel as though you don't have the energy to do anything, but here's the catch-22: the more you exercise, the more energy it'll give you. So the key, as we've said before, is to just do it as best you can. We promise you that if you keep at it on a regular schedule, you will feel the benefits as listed above.

Write it down on your calendar so that it becomes a must-do task, rather than an extracurricular activity that you may or may not get to by the end of the day. Choose a time when you know you have the best chance of committing, such as first thing in the morning or on your lunch break or right before dinner.

Some suggestions for moderate exercise:

- Walking
- Yoga
- Swimming
- Cycling
- Dancing (in the privacy of your home!)
- Low-impact aerobics
- Rebounding (on a mini trampoline)
- Tennis or badminton
- Playing catch with a friend or your dog
- Frisbee
- Household chores like raking leaves/mowing the lawn/vacuuming/washing the car

My favorite exercise is walking, but sometimes people are even embarrassed to do that. I would recommend, if you are serious, to gather the courage, find a workout buddy, and hold each other accountable. Maybe even visit structured classes of some sort together.

We think the tiny shift in the way you view the exercise and the reasons you are doing it in the first place can really launch your recovery from sugar addiction.

Exercise is more important than you think and much more important for recovery from sugar addiction than for burning calories.

MEDITATION

Meditation is all the rage these days with Fortune 500 companies, the Healthcare Industry, our public schools systems, colleges and universities, and even tech companies like Google, Apple, and Facebook.

We try to steer clear of advising people on their spiritual life here at SugarAddiction.com, but we do believe it is a necessary part of recovery and one you should cultivate, however it fits into your life. It definitely brings us much peace and comfort, and that intangible thing that we need to move forward.

Benefits of Meditation

Meditation has been practiced for thousands of years and is a very useful tool for cultivating relaxation and a calm mind, as well as for getting know and trust yourself. Meditating will help you learn that you don't have to listen to all that negative self-talk that echoes around your head all day but rather focus on the things that are important.

The benefits of meditation include:

- Gaining a new perspective on stressful situations
- Building skills to manage your stress
- Increasing self-awareness
- Focusing on the present
- Reducing negative emotions
- Calming anxiety
- Relieving depression
- Lowering blood pressure
- Easing pain
- Improving sleep

I literally can't describe to you in words the benefits that a solid meditation practice has brought to my life. There is just a calmness that I feel, even in the face of what seems impossible.

If it's time to change your life by changing the way you eat, then it's time to work on the mind and the thoughts that got you here. A solid meditation practice can get you to your goals quicker.

How to Meditate

Meditation is very simple: you just sit quietly and focus your attention away from your thoughts, generally on your breathing. There are many different ways to meditate, such as:

- **Guided meditation** – where you visualize images of places or scenarios that you find relaxing. Generally this is easiest when you are guided by a teacher or tape.
- **Mantra meditation** – where you repeat a word or phrase to prevent distracting thoughts. This can also be done by following a tape.
- **Mindfulness or breath meditation** – where you practice increased awareness by focusing on your breathing. When thoughts or emotions come up, you simply acknowledge them and let them go.
- **Transcendental meditation** – where you repeat a personally assigned mantra, such as a word, sound or phrase, in a specific way by a certified teacher. This usually costs a fee.

Mindfulness or breath meditation is probably the easiest to get going on right away. Choose a time, generally first thing in the morning or last thing at night, close your eyes, and sit comfortably for anywhere from 5-20 minutes (or longer, but it's best to start small). That's it. You'll find that your mind races and jumps and thinks and shouts and sings and provokes, etc. Your only job is to continue to sit there until your time is up. Every time a thought comes into your head, just gently pull your mind back to focus on your breathing.

YOU CAN'T DO THIS ALONE: OUR SUPPORT GROUP

No one wants to go through recovery alone, and that's okay to admit because, the truth is, you can't do it alone. Human beings are herd animals. We thrive in groups. We belong in groups. We are sometimes our own worst enemies. If we could do this alone we already would have, right?

I can hear what you're probably saying now: "But I don't want to go to meetings, I hate those stupid meetings!" Okay. We're cool with that. But you do have to find someone, at least one person, who understands *exactly* where you are, what you are doing to yourself, and your plan to walk out of it. You have to be honest with this person and honest with yourself.

Family and friends are great, but they've been around you for awhile and know you as you are; they're used to you that way and, quite frankly, most people don't like change. They might not be as supportive as you'd like them to be, or need them to be. That's not something to blame them for; it's just the nature of most relationships. You also might not be as open to being honest with them.

So it's up to you to find the support of people who can be objective, who will not be afraid to be honest with you, who will call you on your BS if they need to, whom you can be totally honest with and not be afraid of being judged. Most of all, they need to *understand* your very real dependency. If your family and friends don't share your dependency/addiction, they're less likely to "get it" and therefore less likely to be able to help you.

To help support you we have opened a [private Facebook group](#) for all the folks who have downloaded this book (and read this far). In the group you can be as active or passive as you like. You can just lurk and observe or you can dive in and make friends with people all over the globe who are actively participating in their own recovery from Sugar Addiction. Your participation will always be anonymous. No one will know of your participation unless you tell them. (It's very cool new technology - thanks Facebook!)

Successful People Never Do It Alone

Whether a person is successful financially, in their career, as new parents, or health-wise, they all lean on a support group of some kind. Even the big names like Steve Jobs, Oprah, and Bill Gates. That's how they get to the top of their game. They built a team of experts, advisors, and others with whom they can get guidance, advice, feedback, and encouragement. Richard Branson, entrepreneur and founder of Virgin Group, has said that the reason he's successful is because of his team.

A Word On 12-Step Programs

They could be an integral part of your recovery. Our opinion about 12-step programs is based on 30 years of attendance at meetings worldwide. Having a support group and a program to follow is essential. You may be aware of OA (Overeaters Anonymous), which is the largest of these programs. OA does not have a defined eating plan and its members get to "name their own abstinence."

Many people in OA define their abstinence as we do and we believe abstinence as we have defined it is critical to your success.

But we'd like to recommend two other 12-step programs that do define abstinence in the same way we do: one is FAA (Food Addicts Anonymous) and the other is Food Addicts in Recovery.

CEA-How and The Greysheeters are two other groups but are very small. Of the list above I would suggest Food Addicts in Recovery if you are inclined that way.

It doesn't matter what form of support you get, as long as you reach out to a safe group (and a safe group can be defined as just ONE other person at first!) or therapist to guide and travel with you in your journey.

There are many ways to succeed, but doing it alone is not one of them.

Start in our Facebook group. We discuss absolutely everything you need to recover and from there you can meet others and pair off into smaller groups that work together, play together and recover together.

Many people just use the Facebook group alone. Not a member yet?
Join us here

CONCLUSION

I've been asked what I hope you, the reader, will get from this book. The answer is two things.

One is hope.

I hope that I have been able to shine the light on this issue just enough for you to feel that there is a possibility that you, too, can be successful in ending your sugar dependency, and that you can see a clear path to serenity and peace around food, a path that others have taken successfully and one you can also travel.

The second thing, and the one I take most seriously as the steward of the site SugarAddiction.com, is that I want you know, deep in your being, *that you are not alone.*

It is well known that folks like us are "isolators" and that we tend to hide our eating and so we tend to hide ourselves.

Until now our entire life has been spent in a prison of isolation and the cure is simply to reverse that pattern of isolation. We were not born with it. Humans are herd animals. We thrive and grow, live and love with others.

It is also well known that one of the cures, if not the primary one, for these types of maladies are mutual aid societies. Groups of like-kind, like-minded people banding together to support each other on the journey.

I want you to know that you have that here. As we grow this site many more resources will be set into place for you to meet with others on this same journey.

Your feedback is incredibly valuable to me and I really wish you, the very small percentage of folks who read this book all the way through, would send me your feedback. Anything really. I have tough skin. I can take criticism and critique as long as it's positive and would help the site serve others. Tell me what you need or would like to see. We are in this together and I see this site as yours with me as the steward. If you've ever thought that you could or would want to help others once you've begun to heal from sugar addiction, then you've come to the right place. Honestly, that's what we're all about.

We can't reach a lot of people unless the people who change and get better then help others do the same!

Send me your comments to Michael (at) SugarAddiction.com

Be well,
Michael

Check out the interview from The Kick Sugar Summit and all of the free gifts, tips and tools mentioned at the end of some of the chapters right here.

Made in the USA
Coppell, TX
05 April 2022

76038678R00044